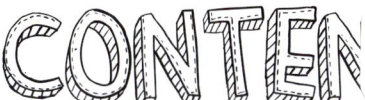

Introduction	4
Safety First	5
Responding to an Emergency	6
Vital Signs	9
Choking	12
Rescue Breathing	13
CPR	14
Pet First Aid	16
Allergic Reactions	16
Back Injuries	18
Bleeding	18
Broken Bones / Fractures	20
Heatstroke	21
Frostbite	22
Poisoning	23
Seizures	24
Shock	25
Bee & Other Insect Stings	27
Upset Tummy	28
Pet First Aid Kit	29
Glossary	30
About the Co-Author/Editor	31
About the Co-Author/Publisher	32
Rescuer's Notes	33

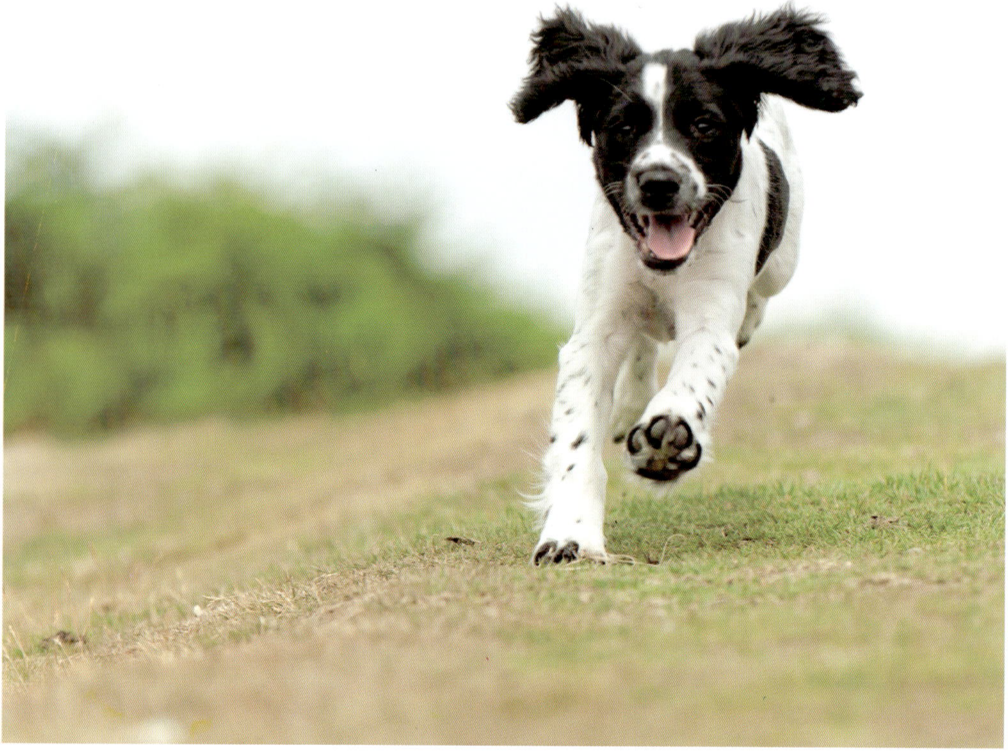

INTRODUCTION

This book is a quick reference to teach you (if you are age 8 or older), what to do if your dog or cat needs help. You will discover ways to keep both yourself and your pets safe, how to find help, what supplies to keep on hand and what to tell your parents in case of an emergency (Imagine being able to tell your parents what to do – how cool is that?!).

We urge you to involve your parents in a **Pet First Aid & CPR Class** so that your family is properly equipped with these life-saving skills.

You are encouraged to practice on a **Rescue Critters!**® CeePeR mannikin or a stuffed toy so that you'll be ready to help when help is needed! Just remember…always practice Safety First.

SAFETY FIRST

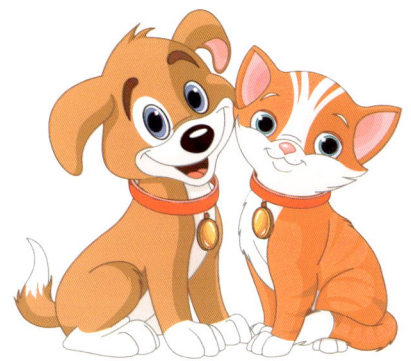

The first and most important thing to do is **STAY SAFE!** **STOP, LOOK, LISTEN & TELL** come next.

STOP means STOP right where you are.
If you run to help a pet in trouble, you might fall and hurt yourself, and then you won't be able to help the pet.

LOOK around you and notice anything that could cause harm, but **DO NOT TOUCH** other animals, anything sharp or broken, spilled liquids, electric wires or anything unusual or dangerous. Also pay attention to your pet's body language – Are his ears back or tail between his legs? Has your cat pulled her whiskers back against her cheeks? Is the fur standing up on your pet's neck or back, or is kitty's tail all puffed up? Is the animal showing his teeth? Any of these things could mean your pet is scared and could bite…even you, so beware!

LISTEN for sounds such as growling, barking or hissing from your pet, traffic noise or even the sound of gas leaking or an electric sizzle kind of sound. This information could let you know where the problem is coming from and help you provide an adult with useful information. If the animal is growling, slowly back away, watching him but do not stare directly into his eyes which could appear threatening.

TELL your parents or another grown-up you know that there is trouble and your pet needs help.

Responding To An Emergency

Be Prepared:

Know where your nearest 24 Hour Emergency Veterinary Hospital is located. Ask your parents to drive you there now (before you need it), so that you will all know exactly where it is and what services they provide.

Keep your Veterinarian's phone number by the phone or programmed into it.

Have a well-stocked Pet First-Aid Kit on hand (see page 29).

Make sure your pet **ALWAYS** has an easy-to-read Identification Tag on his collar and is micro-chipped. Check with your parents that the micro-chip has been registered with your address and phone number so that if Fido or Fluffy gets lost, someone will know who to call to make sure your pet gets home to you!

Safely Approach An Injured Animal:

Remember to **STOP, LOOK & LISTEN** so that you can **TELL** your parent or other adult that something is not quite right.

Always approach an injured animal carefully – remember to listen for sounds and watch their body language.

Talk softly to the animal as you get near and if he appears friendly, offer the back of your hand for him to sniff before slowly scratching under his chin to gain his trust. *Never pat any animal on the head!* Raising your hand might make the dog or cat think you are going to slap or hit him. If he starts to growl or back away, stop what you are doing.

Muzzle & Restrain:

Even your best friend might bite when he is in pain or afraid, so with the help of an adult, you may need to muzzle & restrain your pet to look at an injury or take him to the Vet.

A self-made muzzle using a 1" wide strip of soft fabric.

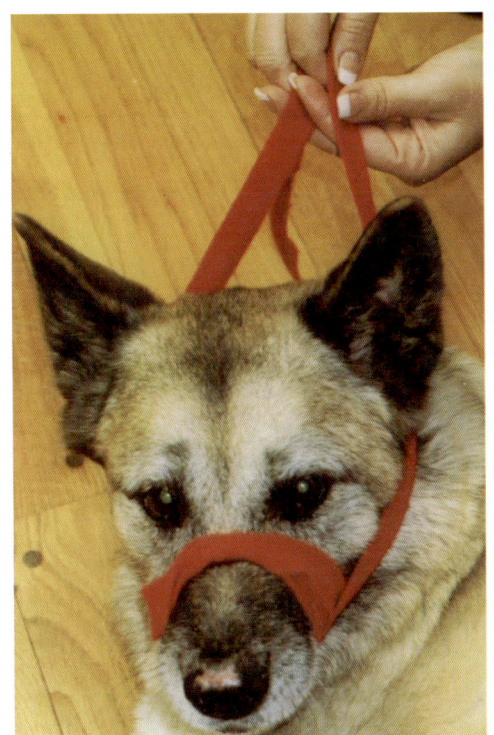

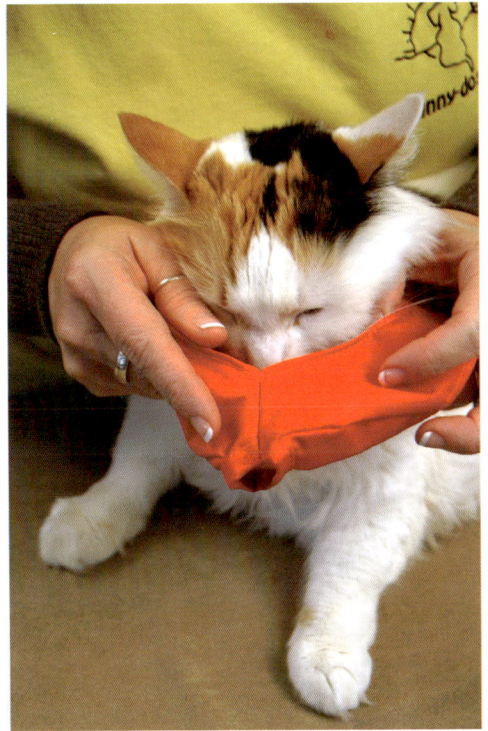

A store bought muzzle for your cat.

Restraining a pet can just mean getting him in a safe environment. If he can walk, try to get your cat or small dog to go into a bathroom where you can close the door. Sometimes they feel more secure if you wrap them in a towel.

If the animal is outside, get him on a leash. If you don't restrain an injured animal in one of these ways, he could run away and be harmed further.

Next you may need to muzzle your pet. **Don't worry** – a properly applied muzzle will not hurt your cat or dog and is not cruel. Use a store-bought one that is the right size, or make one yourself out of a leash or fabric that is soft and about 1" wide (gauze roll from your first aid kit, torn up strip of sheet). Do not use something narrow that might cut his snout when pulled tight – no rope, string, shoe laces, wire or cord of any type.

Make a loop first and drop it over your pet's snout. Pull ends tight and then cross under his chin.

Finally, bring around back of neck and tie off in a bow – never a knot in case you need to remove the muzzle quickly due to breathing or other difficulties. Never leave a pet alone when he has a muzzle on!

Transport:

Call the Veterinarian's office or Animal Emergency Center to let them know you will be bringing in your pet and give them as much information as possible.

If your pet cannot walk, have your parents carefully carry him or lift him on a board if they think he may have broken a bone.

Have your parent or guardian safely drive you and your four-legged friend to the **Vet or Animal ER.**

VITAL SIGNS

Breathing/ Respiration:

Look, Listen & Feel for breathing...

Look... Is your pet's chest moving up and down as he breathes in and out?

Listen... Can you hear your pet breathe? Is there a "gasp" as he takes in air or a "puff" as he lets the air out?

Feel... Can you feel his chest moving or feel air leaving his mouth? If you can, count how many times he either breathes in or out for 30 seconds and then double that number.

Normal Respiration

Large Dogs	10 – 30 breaths per minute
Small Dogs & Cats	20 – 40 breaths per minute

If not, you may need to breathe for your pet by giving him Rescue Breathing.

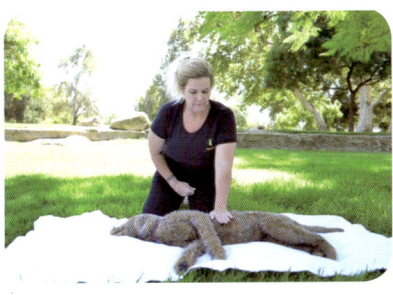

Place your hand on the side of the chest to feel for breathing.

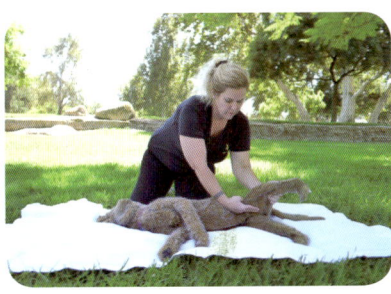

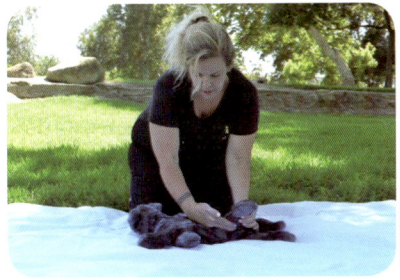

Check for a pulse at the Femoral Artery, just inside the thigh on either hind leg.

Pulse:
The pulse is the movement of blood through an artery. It lets you know if your dog or cat's heart is working.

For large dogs, feel the ***Femoral Artery*** which is located on your dog's inner thigh. Place your index and middle fingers where his rear leg meets his body and see if you feel a pulse similar to what you'd feel at your own wrist. Count for 30 seconds and then double that number.

For small dogs and cats, sometimes the ***Apical Pulse*** is easier to check. Place your hand on the animal's chest just behind the shoulder – where his elbow touches his chest if you move it back slightly.

Normal Pulse Rates
Large Dogs	60 – 160 beats per minute
Small Dogs & Cats	120 – 220 beats per minute

Temperature:
To take your pet's temperature, you'll need help from an adult, but a digital thermometer works best. The rectum is located beneath the base of the tail. Be sure to put some water-based lubricant on the tip of the thermometer. Insert the thermometer no more than one inch into the rectum.
Normal Temperature for Dogs & Cats
　　　100.4°F – 102.5°F or 38°C – 39.1°C

Capillary Refill Time (CRT):

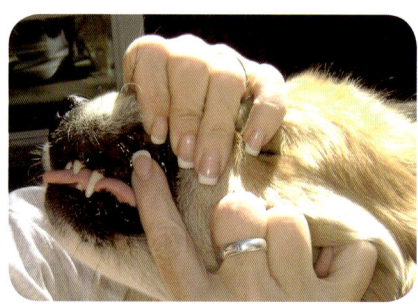

By checking your pet's CRT, you can find out how well the blood is moving through his body. In other words, you are checking his circulation!

Only if your pet will allow, gently lift his lip with your fingers as shown in the picture and then using a finger on your other hand, press his gums right above the teeth until the gum turns lighter.

Release the pressure and count how long it takes for the color of the gums (generally pink) to return.

If it takes more than 2 seconds for the color to return, your pet needs to see the Vet immediately! We call this condition **Shock** (refer to page 25). As you quickly transport your pet, you should cover him with a sheet to keep him warm, and keep his hind legs elevated on a pillow to make sure blood is flowing to his heart.

Hydration:

Pets are 70% water, just like humans and the planet Earth! They need plenty of fresh water all day long.

Only if the pet will allow you to safely lift his lip, feel his gums.

If they are sloppy wet, he is well hydrated.

If his gums are dry or sticky, encourage him to drink or have him checked out by his Veterinarian.

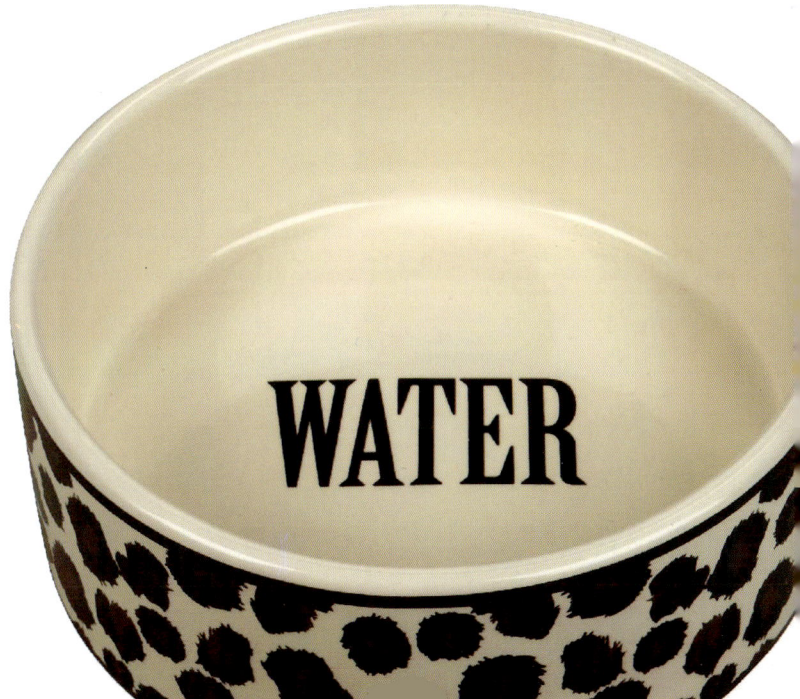

CHOKING

Choking is common with pets. Don't panic! Most of the time animals will clear their own airway by coughing, but if they don't or you can't get a breath in when you try to do Rescue Breathing, you may then need to clear their airway for them!

If the pet is Conscious (meaning awake/alert)...

Get behind him and gently place your fist in the soft part of his belly, right in the middle of his stomach.

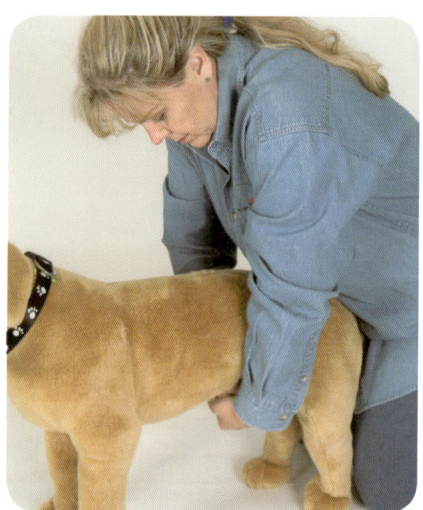 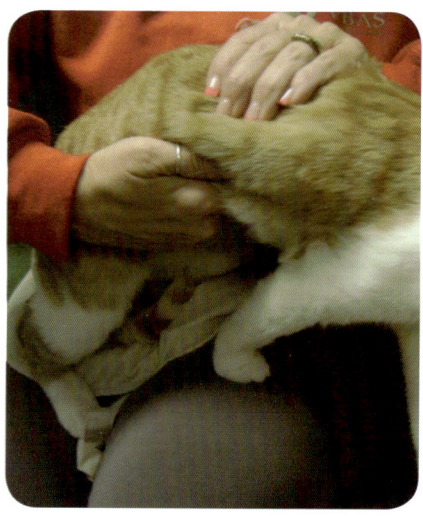

Performing abdominal thrusts on a dog (left) and a cat (right)

Wrap your other hand around him like you're giving him a big hug and then pull forward towards your own chest 5 times (his back must be against your chest to do this properly). This is called **Abdominal Thrusts.**

If this is a cat or small dog, instead of your whole fist, just use the tips of a couple fingers and hold the pet's back with your other hand. This way you are pressing your finger tips up towards your hand as your fist may be too big to use on a small pet.

Hopefully this will remove what is stuck in his airway!

If the pet is Unconscious (not awake but not just sleeping)...

Look, Listen & Feel for breathing (page 9).

If he's not breathing, give your pet **Rescue Breathing** (see section below).

If your breaths are not going in, you will need to clear the airway first. With an adult's help, look inside pet's mouth to see if there is an object that needs removing and do so. You may need to gently pull the tongue forward. Then proceed with Rescue Breathing.

RESCUE BREATHING

Rescue Breathing is when you have to breathe for your dog or cat because they are not breathing on their own. You should do rescue breathing **only** when they are not breathing but when they do have a pulse.

Rescue Breathing is also known as **Mouth-to-Snout Resuscitation!**
Look, Listen & Feel for breathing.

If pet is not breathing...

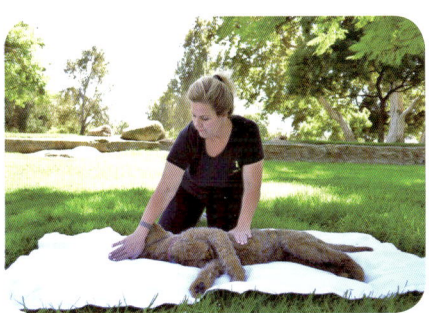

Pull back on the chin to open the airway.

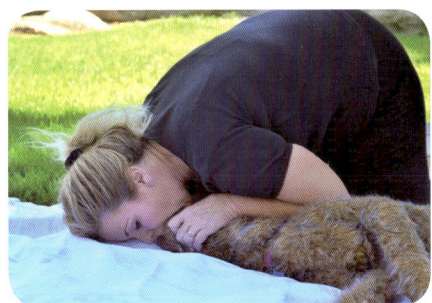

Deliver two slow breaths directly into the nostrils just until you see the chest rise (Mouth-to-Snout).

This is an emergency, but stay calm and lay pet on his side.

Gently push his chin upward (keeping side of pet's face on the ground) to stretch out his throat area and open his airway.

Close his mouth and give two breaths into his nostrils, wrapping your lips around the end of his snout. Blow only hard enough that you begin to see his chest rise.

Check for a Pulse (page 10)

If there is a pulse, continue Rescue Breathing and after every 10 breaths or 30 seconds, recheck his pulse.

If there is not a pulse, begin CPR (see section below).

If air is not going in, something may be caught in his airway. Go to the Choking section (page 12).

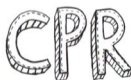

CPR (Cardio Pulmonary Resuscitation) is performed when a dog or cat is not breathing and has no pulse. This is an emergency situation! Stay calm so that you can focus on helping your pet.

If after you've given your dog or cat Rescue Breathing (page 13), you determine there is no pulse, you need to start **Chest Compressions!**

With pet laying on his right side on a hard surface (floor, ground or table – not your lap or a sofa), gently pull his front left leg back until his elbow touches his chest. This marks the spot for you to place your hands or fingers for Chest Compressions.

For medium to large dogs, use the heel of your hand with the other hand on-top of it – fingers locked – to compress 2-3 inches.

For cats and small dogs, use the tips of 2 fingers to compress ½ inch – 1 inch. You can also wrap one hand or both around a small animal's chest to do compressions.

No matter what size animal, do 30 Compressions and then give 2 Rescue Breaths and repeat.

After every 4 rounds (approximately 2-3 minutes), recheck the pulse. If there is still no pulse, get your parents or other adult ready to drive you and your pet to the Vet as soon as possible while you continue **CPR.**

If you get a pulse, check if your pet is now also breathing on his own. If so, get him to the Vet monitoring his breathing all the way there. If not, continue Rescue Breaths...

On a dog:

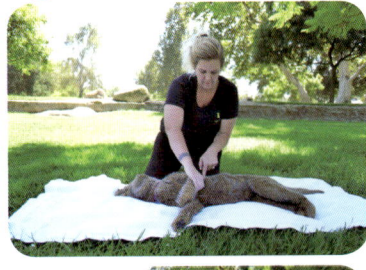

Gently pull back the elbow until it touches the chest to locate the heart.

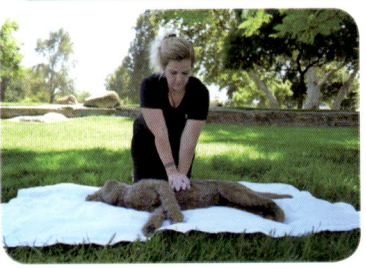

Position the heel of your hand in this location, lock fingers and elbows and get ready to...

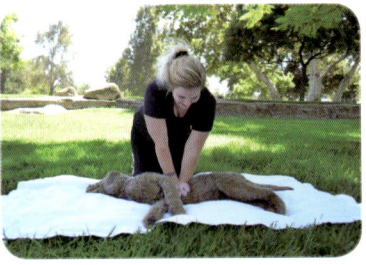

Compress 1/3 the width of the chest at a rate of 30 compressions to 2 breaths, rechecking the pulse every 4 rounds.

On a cat:

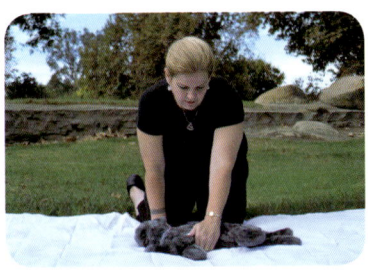

Feel for the heartbeat.

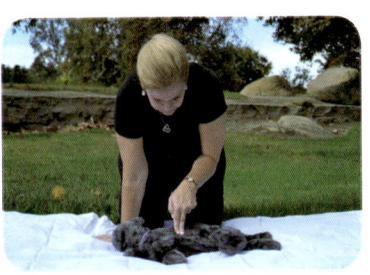

Two finger chest compressions method.

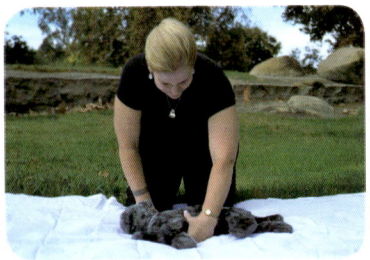

Wrap chest compressions method.

PET FIRST AID

Just like in the first part of this book, remember that **SAFETY IS NUMBER 1!** Stop, Look & Listen, wear medical gloves (Pet First Aid Kit page 29) when dealing with wounds or cleaning up after your pet, and have your dog or cat checked by your Veterinarian whenever you think something is not quite right.

Also, make sure you take him to the Vet for annual check-ups so that problems can be caught early! It's also a good idea to sit down with your pet once a week and just look him over checking for fleas, ticks, cuts or scrapes, check his vitals and feel for any lumps, bumps or anything out of the ordinary. That will help make you your pet's best friend!

ALLERGIC REACTIONS

Sometimes dogs and cats become allergic to food, the grass, insect stings, medication, laundry soap or just about anything and their body reacts.

Signs Include:
Difficulty breathing
Swelling and/or pain
Constantly licking paws or the same body part over and over.
Redness
Vomiting or Diarrhea
Shock (page 25) This is an emergency situation!

What to Do:
Look, Listen & Feel for breathing
Do Rescue Breathing or CPR if needed (pages 13-15)
Apply a cold pack or ice wrapped in a towel to any swelling for short periods of time.
Call your Veterinarian for advice on giving medications.
Take your pet to the Vet if condition worsens or if your Veterinarian suggests.

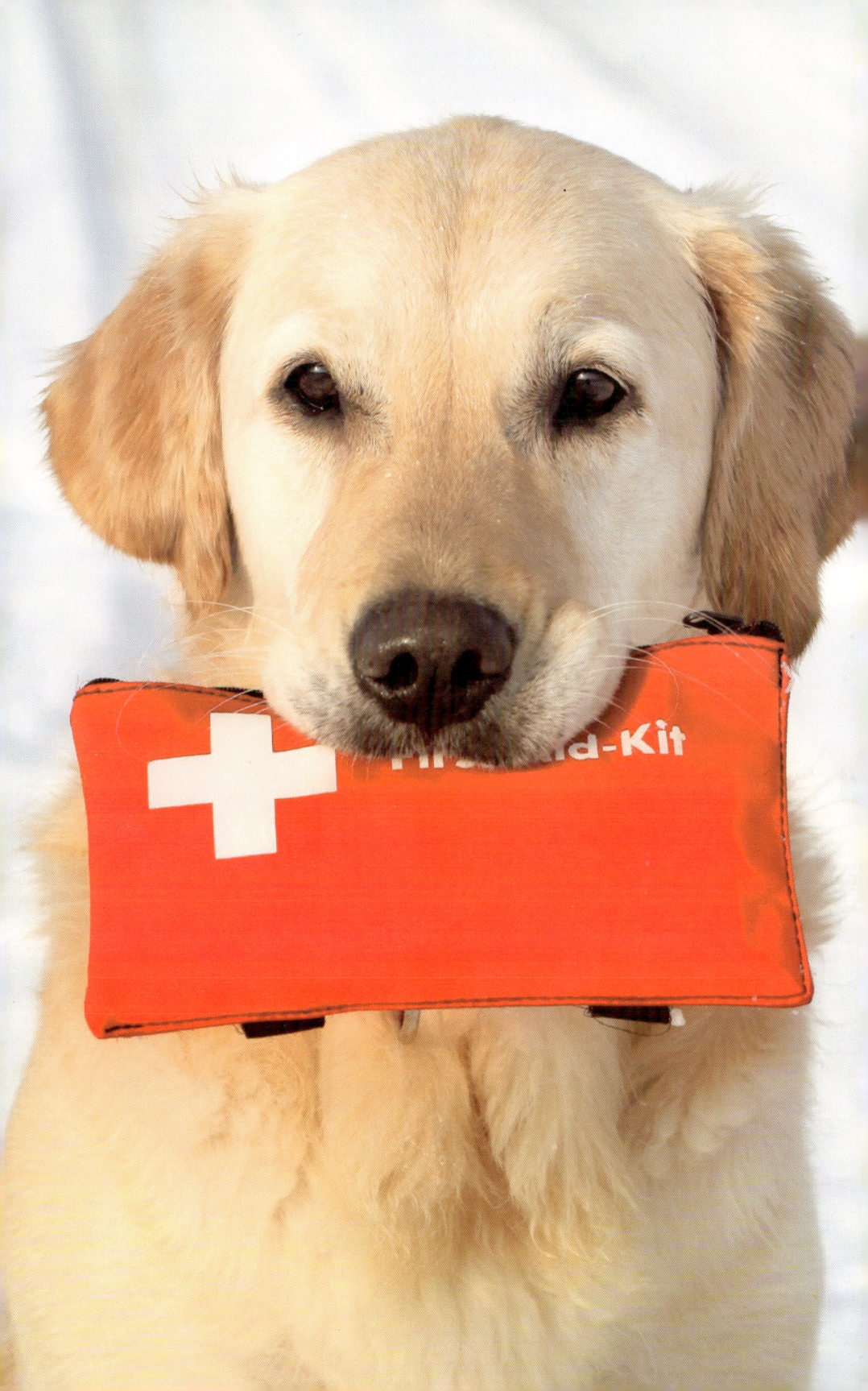

BACK INJURIES

If your pet has been hit by a car, been dropped, falls from a wall or window or has been tossed during an animal fight, you can suspect back or neck injuries and you must move him carefully so as not to cause further injury.

Signs Include:
Can't stand up or unable to use legs
May try but drags their hind legs
Seems to be in pain

What to Do:
Look, Listen & Feel for breathing and do Rescue Breathing/CPR if needed.

Muzzle your pet – Safety first!
Gently slide pet onto a board or other flat surface. The board needs to be bigger than your pet and strong enough to hold his weight. You will need an adult to help and maybe even two adults to carry each end depending on the size of the animal.

    Piece of plywood
    Ironing Board or Surf Board
    Lid off a plastic storage box or cookie sheet for a small pet

Call your Veterinarian's Office to let them know you are coming and have an adult drive you and your pet there as soon as possible.

Strap the hips and shoulders of your pet to the board using a triangular bandage, strips of sheet or even leashes if they are long enough.

BLEEDING

Animals, like humans, sometimes bleed a little and sometimes bleed a lot.

Signs Include:
Blood on the skin
Blood coming from the nose, mouth or other part of the body

What to Do:

Muzzle if pet seems to be in pain so that you will not get bitten when trying to help.

For small amounts of blood (small cut or scrape), go to your Pet First Aid Kit and clean the wound with the eye wash (purified water). Pat it dry and cover with a bandage until an adult or your Veterinarian determines if any medicine is needed.

For lots of blood, you must stop the bleeding!

Check breathing, pulse and for Shock! (pages 9-11)

Put on medical gloves and apply direct pressure to the wound with gauze squares out of your **Pet First Aid Kit** (page 29). Never remove the first bandage you apply, but if you need more gauze…add it on top of the first layer. If you remove that first layer of gauze square, you break the blood clot that is trying to form and allow bacteria to get into the wound.

If the bleeding isn't stopping, place a pillow or rolled up towel underneath the part of your pet's body that is bleeding (elevation).

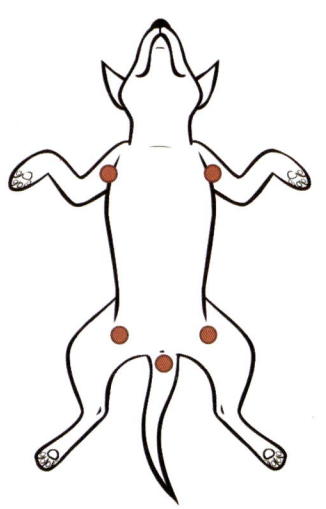

If the bleeding still doesn't stop and is on a leg or tail, apply pressure to the corresponding pressure point while you continue to appy direct pressure to the wound. Pressure points are major arteries and are located inside each leg and at the base of the tail. By pressing on them, you slow down the blood flowing out of the wound.

Wrap gauze squares with gauze roll and secure with tape.

Call your Veterinarian and have an adult drive you and your pet there immediately.

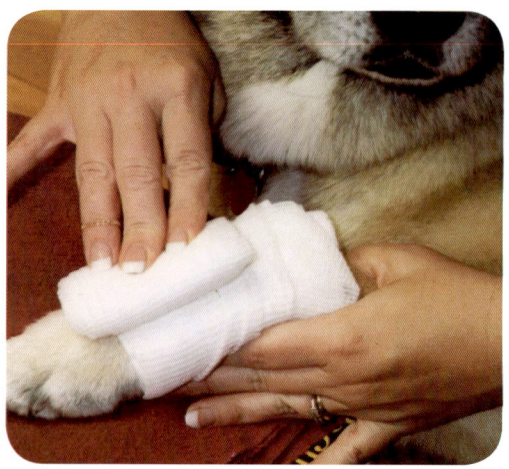
Applying direct pressure.

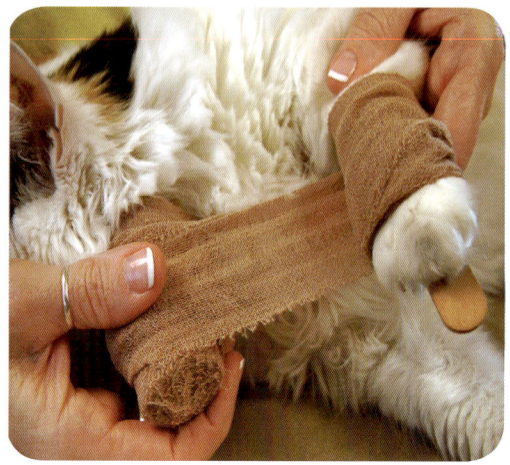
Bandaging a wound using a popsicle stick as a splint.

BROKEN BONES/FRACTURES

Your dog or cat can break a bone when they fall, are dropped, get in a fight with another animal or are in a car accident. Breaks can hurt a whole lot!

Signs Include:

Swelling or deformity
Leg facing the wrong direction or dangling
Pet limps or cries in pain
Bone visibly sticks out through skin

What to Do:

Check breathing, pulse and **CRT** (pages 9-11).

Muzzle & restrain your pet for safety (pages 6-8). Keep pet as calm as possible and prevent them from moving.

If you see the bone, don't move it. Cover with gauze squares or a clean towel to stop bleeding.

Make a splint! A splint keeps your dog or cat's limb from moving and prevents further injury to it. For a medium to large dog, you can use a rolled up magazine or newspaper. For smaller pets, a popsicle stick, unsharpened pencil, even a wooden spoon or small stick will work. Hold the splint in place with the triangular bandage or stretchy adhesive tape in your Pet First Aid Kit. Just make sure you do not wrap it too tightly – swelling or coldness below the splint or even when bandaging a wound could be a danger sign!

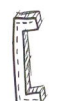 *Call your Veterinarian to let him know you and your pet are on your way and get adult transportation.*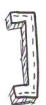

HEATSTROKE

Pets get overheated when left in a parked car, when exercising on hot days, on cold days when the heat is turned up high, or anytime they don't have enough water and their body temperature is too high. Heatstroke can be very serious!

Signs Include:

Heavy panting or difficulty breathing
Bright red gums, tongue and inner eye lids
Foaming around the mouth or Dehydrated (dry or sticky gums)
Pet is slow, inactive or collapses
104°F/40°C or higher Temperature

What to Do:

Get Pet out of hot environment and into a cooler one – shade, tile bathroom or kitchen floor, in front of a fan or car air conditioner.

Cool dog or cat off from the paws up to his belly in a tub of water (not ice water). Do not get him wet up to his neck as that will cool him off too quickly. Keep water running but drain open, and never leave a pet alone in water.

Wipe rubbing alcohol (from your Pet First Aid Kit) onto the pads of their feet and the inner flaps of his ears. This cools off the blood in these areas which then travels throughout the body.

Get adult assistance and take your pet's temperature.
If it is 104°F or higher, or if your pet seems to be in distress…Call your Veterinarian and get an adult to drive you and your pet there right away.

FROSTBITE

Just like an animal can get too hot, a dog or cat can get too cold and this can also be life-threatening!

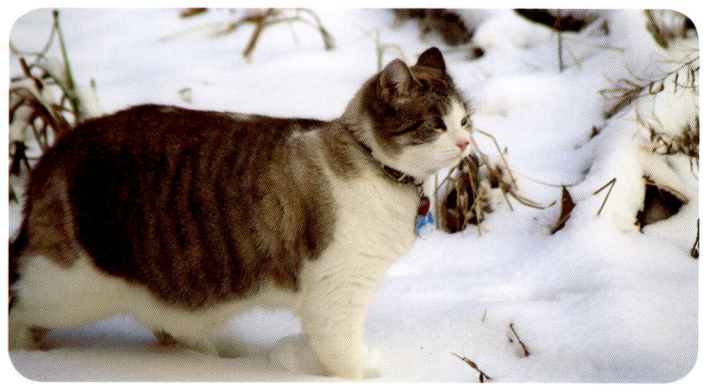

Signs Include:
Pet may cry when trying to walk on paws.
Paws, nose, tail (whatever part is too cold) may feel hard to the touch – it is frozen.
Skin may be pale or bluish (if you can see it through the fur) but then turns dark.

What to Do:
Get pet out of the cold and into a warmer environment – inside! Do not rub the frozen area – it will be extremely painful to your pet. Get them in a tub with room temperature water running on them (drain open so that it does not fill up) and never leave him alone.

Tumble a towel on the "warm" cycle in the dryer for a few moments and wrap animal in it. If you have low-sodium chicken broth, warm it and see if your pet will drink some to warm him from the inside out.

[*Call your Veterinarian and get your pet there quickly.*]

POISONING

Many things can poison your pet. Some he may ingest (eat or drink), some poisons he could breathe in through his nostrils and others can be absorbed through the pads of his paws and then ingested when he licks and grooms himself.

Do your best to keep dangerous items off the floor and out of paws reach!

Pet Poisons Include:

Medications not prescribed by your Veterinarian
Car fumes
Various plants
Chemicals found in your house and yard (antifreeze, cleaners, insecticides, fertilizers to name a few)
Foods such as coffee, chocolate, grapes & raisins, onions, Macadamia & other nuts
Anything out of the trash including moldy food
Overdose of flea powders, flea collars and dips
Human medicines (aspirin for instance)
Artificial Sweeteners

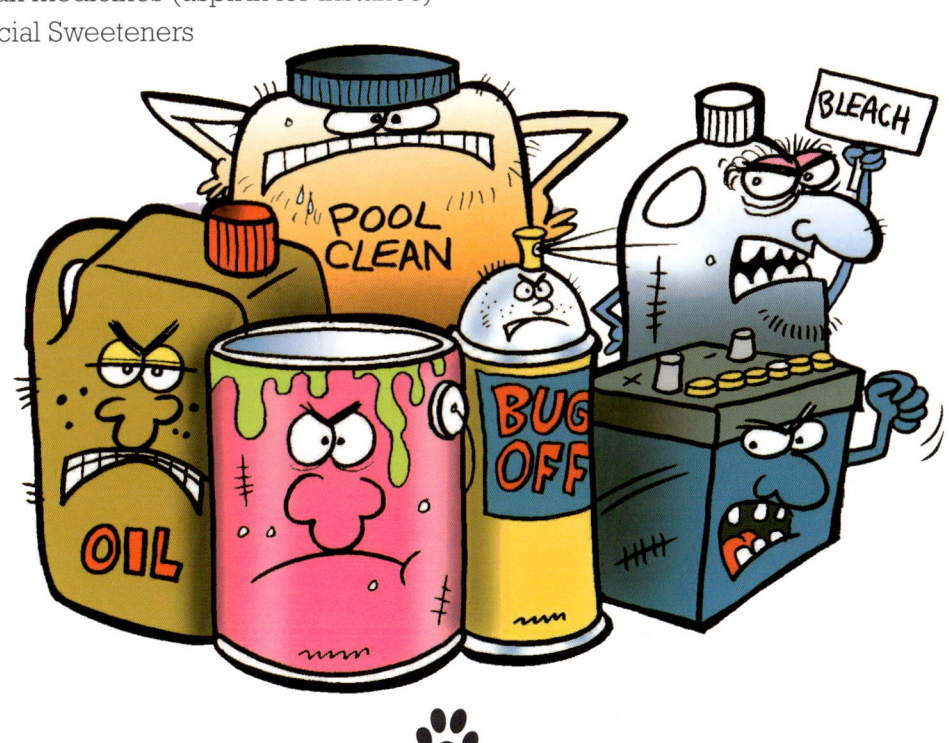

Signs Include:
Vomiting or Diarrhea
Breathing unusual or not at all
Fast or slow pulse
Seizures (see section below)
Bleeding from unusual places (nose, eyes, etc)
Drooling more than normal
Bumps or sores around your pet's mouth
Pet is not acting normal (too excited, too tired, doesn't respond)
Unconscious/Collapses

What to Do:
Check breathing, pulse and **CRT** (pages 9-11).

Look around the house – is there an obvious poison your dog or cat has gotten into? Put on your medical gloves and put the poison you find in a plastic bag.

If pet has vomited or had diarrhea, collect that safely in a plastic bag to show the Vet. **Put on your medical gloves!**

Take the poison and your pet quickly to the Veterinarian, calling first that you are on the way, providing the Vet's Office with any information you have: possible poison, how much and when your pet got into it, what his signs are.

SEIZURES

A seizure is a series of uncontrollable muscle contractions. Your dog or cat may shake or stiffen up and twitch. They are unconscious and can't control their movements. Seizures can happen when your pet is poisoned, suffers heatstroke or other injuries or has Cancer or Epilepsy.

Signs Include:
Shaking or stiffness with twitching
Eyes glazed over
Drooling and loss of control of bodily functions (may urinate and defecate while unconscious)

What to Do

Stay away from mouth – your pet has no control over his jaws snapping and could bite you. He may also growl uncontrollably and this can appear threatening to other animals, so keep them in another room.

Do not try to hold him down.

Move furniture and hard objects out of the way so that your pet will not bang himself. You can toss blankets around him but do not touch your dog or cat.

Do prevent him from falling down stairs.

Step back and watch him as you time the seizure (1 minute, 2 minutes, 5 minutes, etc).

Call your Veterinarian's Office with all the details and if this is a first time seizure or more than several minutes, you will probably be asked to bring your pet in.

Quickly look about the house to see if you can detect any poison your pet may have gotten into that could be the cause of the seizure. If you find any, carefully bring it with you.

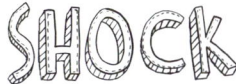

SHOCK

If your pet is in Shock, it means that his tissues and organs are not getting enough Oxygen. Oxygen is pumped by the lungs and travels through the body via the blood stream. Therefore Shock can be caused by lots of bleeding, poor circulation, dehydration, an allergy, poisoning or heatstroke.

Signs Include:

Pet is unconscious
Tissue (mucus membranes) around eyes and gums is pale
Capillary Refill Time (CRT) is longer than 2 seconds
Extremities are cold (paws, ears)
Breathing is too fast or too slow

What to Do:

Check breathing, pulse and CRT (pages 9-11).

Stop any bleeding (pages 18-19).

Cover dog or cat with a sheet or towel to keep in body heat. If their blood isn't circulating properly, it's like their thermostat isn't working and they can't regulate their temperature.

If there is no bleeding to the pet's head or chest, transport them with a folded blanket under their hind legs to encourage circulation to the heart, lungs and other major organs. If there is bleeding to head or chest, just keep pet flat and get to the Veterinarian **ASAP!**

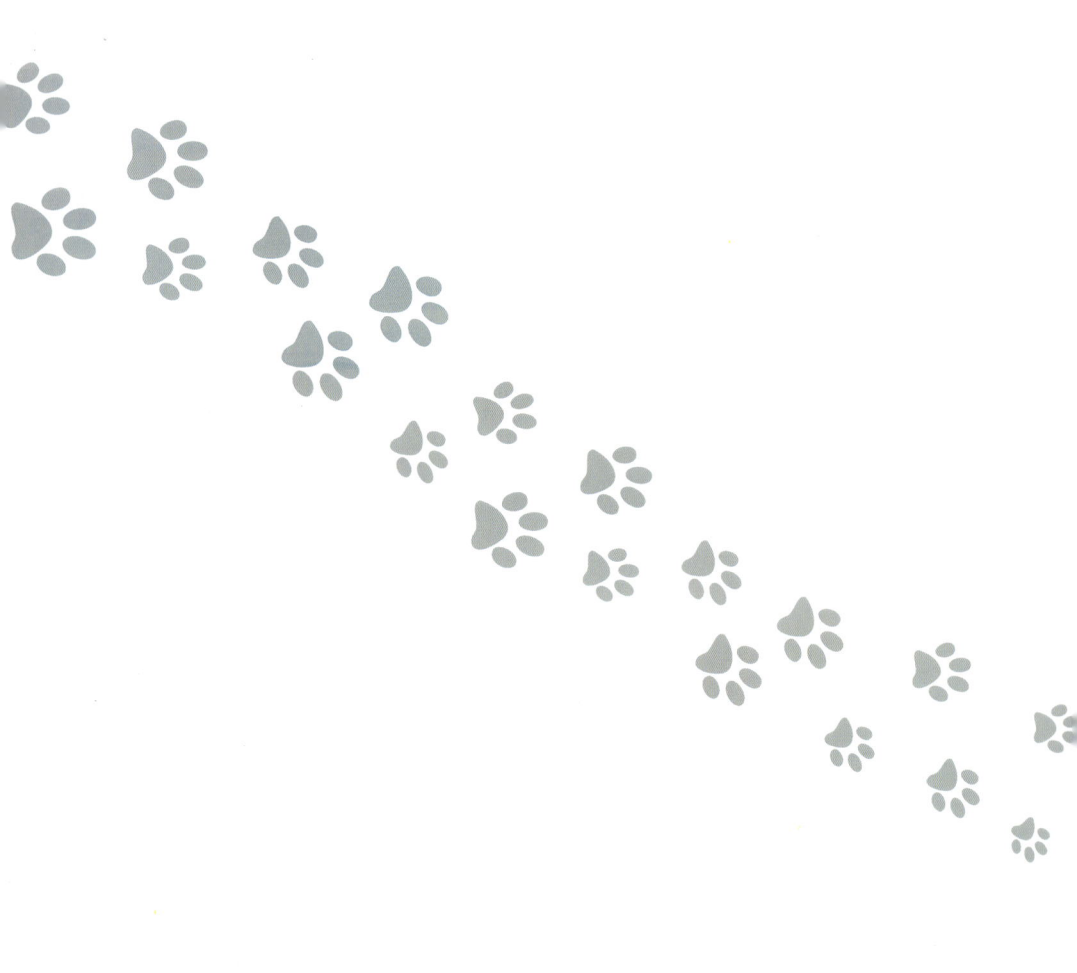

BEE & OTHER INSECT STINGS

Most of the time our dogs and cats get stung on the face as they snap at insects, however they can also step on a bee or sit on an insect so stings can happen on any part of their body.

Signs Include:

Swelling and/or redness
Itchiness – Pet will be rubbing or pawing at area
Possible breathing difficulty

What to Do:

If your pet is having any difficulty breathing, get him immediately to the Veterinarian. A severe allergic reaction from the insect toxin could stop his breathing. For redness and swelling, apply a cold pack 1- 2 minutes then remove for a minute and reapply so as not to give pet frostbite. Continue this "on/off" method for about 15 minutes and hopefully you will see the swelling go down. Call your Veterinarian to see if he suggests giving your pet any medicine.

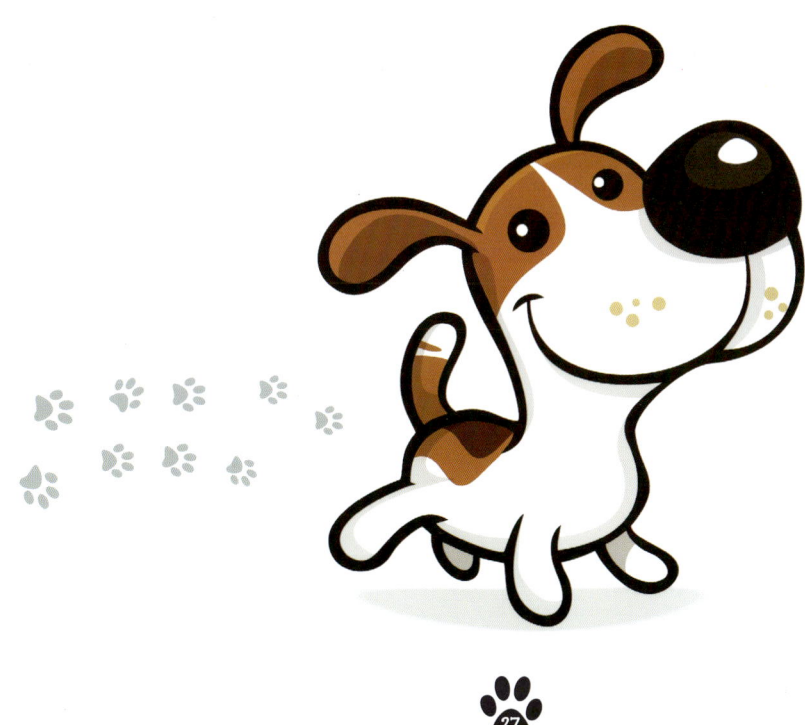

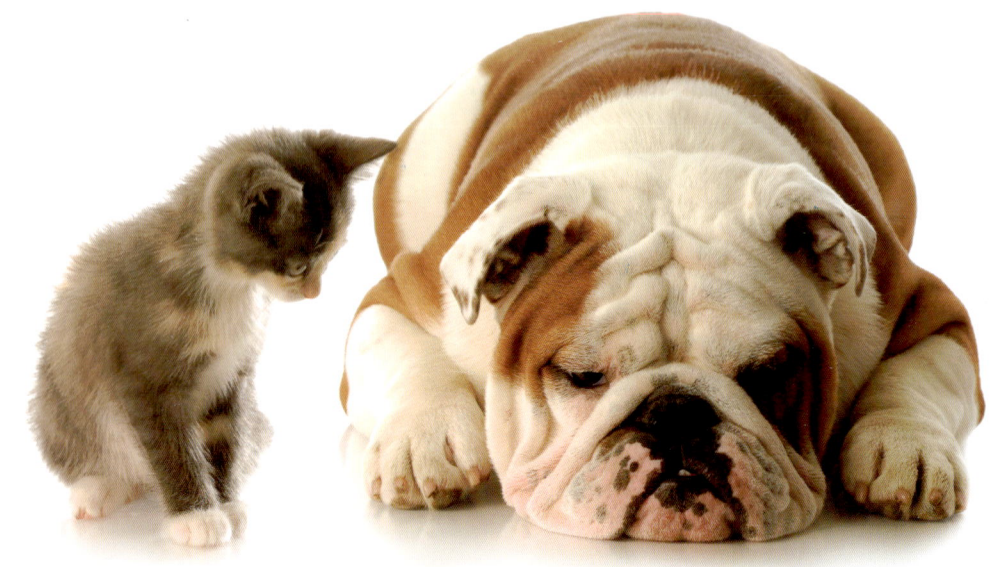

UPSET TUMMY

Just like you, sometimes your dog or cat is not feeling his best. He may have eaten too much, too fast or something he should not have eaten at all.

Signs Include:

Stomach gurgling
Vomiting, Diarrhea

What to Do:

Stop feeding your dog or cat. Whatever is going in is coming back out.

Make sure though that he has plenty of fresh water so that he does not become dehydrated.

Call your Veterinarian to see if he suggests giving your pet any medicine.

If the vomiting or diarrhea has not stopped within 24 hours, or if there is any blood in the vomit or diarrhea, get an adult to take you and your pet to the Veterinarian for a check-up! It might help your Veterinarian if you put on medical gloves and collect some vomit or diarrhea in a plastic bag to bring along for analysis.

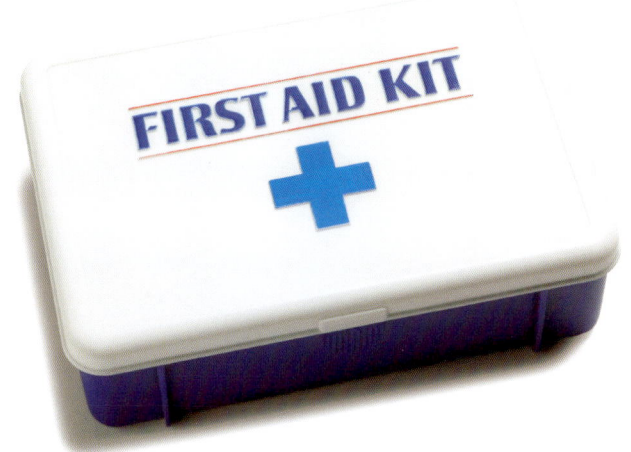

PET FIRST AID KIT

The following items are the basics you should have in your Pet First-Aid Kit. There are always more things you can add, but these are important ones. Also remember that if you use something up you must replace it, and if it expires, you need to get another.

- 4" X 4" Gauze Squares
- 2" Gauze Rolls
- Popsicle Sticks or Tongue Depressors for Splinting
- 2" or 4" Flexible Adhesive Wrap
- 36" or larger Triangular Bandage
- 4 oz bottle of Eye Wash (Saline Solution or Purified Water)
- Rubbing Alcohol
- Cold Pack
- Tweezers
- Blunt-nosed Scissors
- Leash
- Pairs of Medical Gloves
- Clean Towel, Sheet, T-shirt Material
- Plastic zip lock bags to place poisons, vomit or fecal samples in; Picture & Description of your pet in case they get lost; Microchip Number; Vaccination Records; List of known allergies; Important Phone Numbers (Vet, Animal Emergency Center, Local Shelter)

GLOSSARY

Abdominal thrusts - Squeezing the stomach to clear the Airway

Airway - The open part in our throats that lets us breathe

Allergic - A bad reaction to something in our bodies

Apical Pulse - The pulse directly over the heart

Bleeding - When blood exits the body

Capillary Refill Time (CRT) - Shows that there is good circulation. Quick is good (1-2 seconds), longer is bad

Circulation - The word for blood going around in our bodies

Compressions - Pushing down

Conscious - Awake and alert, eyes open

CPR - Cardio (heart) Pulmonary (lungs) Resuscitation (to revive)

Diarrhea - The poops, runs, squirts (you get the idea)

Femoral Artery - The big artery in the inner thigh where you check your dog's or cat's pulse

Heatstroke - Being dangerously hot (temperature of 104F/40C degrees or higher)

Mouth-to-Snout Resuscitation - When you help a pet that cannot breathe by breathing into his nostrils

Poisoning - Something our bodies don't like, very hazardous

Pulse - The heartbeat we feel; the movement of blood through the artery

Oxygen - A natural gas in the air we breath. We need oxygen to live

Rescue Breathing - same as Mouth-to-Snout Resuscitation

Seizures - When a dog/cat becomes unconscious, and his muscles twitch or violently shake uncontrollably

Signs - What you see that may give you a hint that something is wrong

Shock - When not enough blood or oxygen circulates inside the body for the body to function properly

Splint - A rigid material used to keep a limb/leg or back and neck from moving

Unconscious - Not awake, does not respond

Vomiting - Throwing up, barf, blowing chunks (you get the idea)

About the Co-Author/Editor

Denise Fleck was raised by a Great Dane named Ulysses and has spent her life loving animals having been dog mom to eleven and cat mom to one. After a successful career as a Motion Picture Studio Publicist, she followed her heart volunteering at animal shelters and teaching people to take better care of their four-legged friends. In addition to sharing Pet Safety Tips in magazines, on TV and on radio, through her company Sunny-dog Ink, Denise teaches Pet First-Aid & CPR to pet parents, trainers, groomers, pet sitters and any one interested in helping animals live longer, happier, healthier lives. She can also be found instilling her own passion for our furry, feathered, finned & scaled friends in high school students through an after-school Animal Care program she teaches weekly. Denise and her husband Paul currently share their lives with two rescued Japanese Akitas, Haiku & Bonsai. Learn more at www.sunnydogink.com.

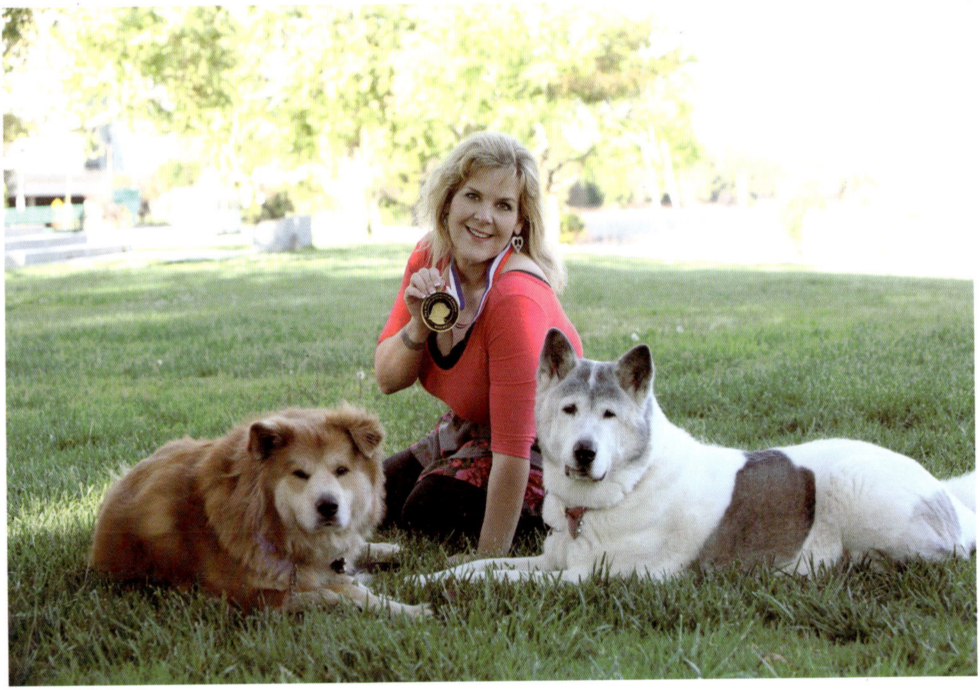

Abour the Co-Author/Publisher

Rescue Critters® was established in 1998. The inspiration came with the realization that there were no simulators available for teaching pet first aid. This idea subsequently led to the development of animal training mannikins catered to the veterinary profession.

From here, Rescue Critters' product range expanded into addressing the needs of the military and Search & Rescue groups to ensure these SAR animals are well taken care of with proper handler training.

Today, our vision is to become the leading provider of these alternative training solutions to veterinary and medical institutions that have been using live animals for practical training and research. We continue to work closely with the military and government agencies in creating products to address their changing requirements.

We believe that with creative innovation, Rescue Critters will be able to refine the educational/training realm, and reduce and replace animal usage to provide a safer and more humane environment for people and animals.
Visit us at www.rescuecritters.com.

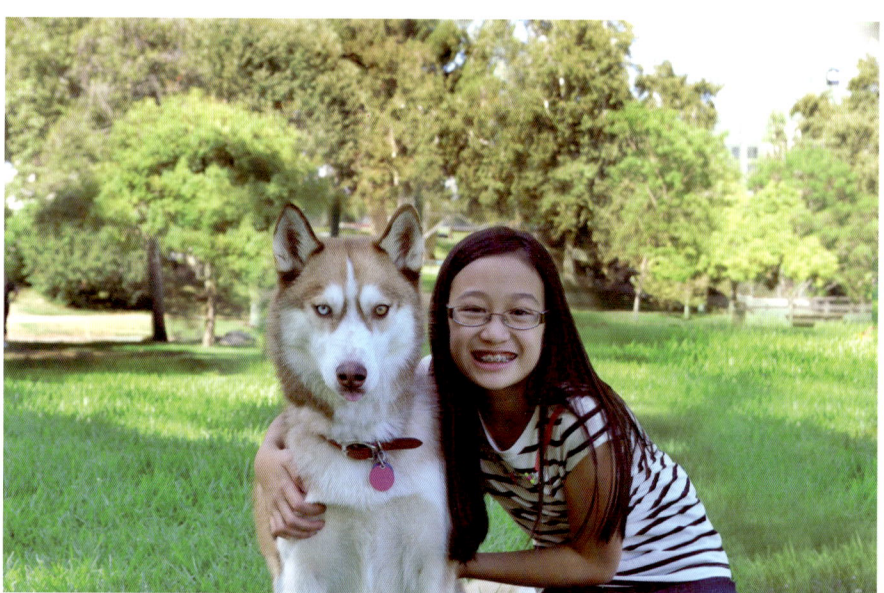

The publisher's daughter, Sophie with photographer Allison Voehringer's pet husky, Patron.

RESCUER'S NOTES

RESCUER'S NOTES